ACID REFLUX DIET

Discover the Secret To Heartburn and Indigestion Cure with the Acid Watcher Diet Plan For Better Gut Relief, GERD, Stomach, and Organ Immunity, Healing, Wellness, and Longevity

Susan Frazier
Daryl Shroder
Jonathan Gioffre

Daryl Wright M.D.

Samin E. Brown

Karen Nosrat M.D.

INTRODUCTION

Acid reflux is one of the most common ailments affecting adults today. This is due to the notion that there are so many contributing factors and catalysts that can spawn its symptoms. As a result, educating oneself on the best ways to care for the symptoms of reflux is paramount for avoiding and overcoming them once they arise.

Evidently, a common refrain for most reflux sufferers is to avoid foods and drinks that are spicy and or fizzy. While these are certainly helpful approaches to take, you are well advised to consider approaches such as increased exercise for maintenance of overall health, avoiding certain exercises altogether if you are already suffering from severe GERD, implementing dietary changes such as limiting coffee intake, cutting back on peppermint and avoiding highly acidic foods.

But acid reflux symptoms are not caused solely by poor dietary choices alone. Indeed, smoking in excess and excess alcohol consumption are also consistent contributing factors that can induce acid reflux symptoms leading to GERD and Barrett's disease. Leveraging the knowledge presented in this book with regard to the specific dietary and lifestyle changes you must implement, along with acquiring a deeper understanding of the particular scientific reasons for acid reflux, will allow for an informed perspective so that your approach to the symptoms presented is equipped with the most up-to-date and effectual information.

When equipped with these strategies and general knowledge concerning acid reflux, you will certainly be at a distinct advantage when you are confronted by the painstaking and, at its most extreme, life-threatening, symptoms of acid reflux.

Table of Contents

PART 1

Chapter 1: Chronic Acid Reflux & Its Serious health Implications

Acid reflux is the result of abundant backflow of acid for your stomach into the esophagus. Anatomically, when your lower esophageal sphincter (LES) becomes weakened by, among many causal factors, continually consuming a high diet, acid can flow back into your esophagus causing acid reflux. Consequently, there are numerous symptoms that are spawned by acid reflux including, most notoriously, heartburn and indigestion. While high acidity in the gut is common for everybody and is often devoid of serious health concerns if occurring on a minimal basis, serious health concerns can develop if high acidity can persist for a prolonged period of time. If left unattended and without measures of control put in place, in many instances, these health issues will lead to hospitalization or even death.

In the most serious cases, chronic long-term heartburn, known as Gastroesophageal Reflux Disease (GERD), Barett's esophagus and esophageal problems can arise due to uncontrolled and unaddressed chronic acidity. Some of these most serious ailments are the remnants of years of neglecting the symptoms of acid reflux, particularly after big meals. Over time, the backflow of acid from your stomach damages your esophagus causing erosion of the layers lining the walls of the organ. This inflammation often leads to very painful swelling in esophagus called esophagitis and is accompanied by a painful swallowing feeling. In addition, esophageal ulcers are the most common ailment of an inflamed esophagus. In fact, GERD is the main cause of these ulcers in the lining of the esophagus. Moreover, painful swallowing, nausea, chest pain contribute to a lack of sleep which perpetuates many of these symptoms simplify virtue of that fact that your body is not getting the required rest to overcome these symptoms. As soon as these symptoms arise, be sure to consult a doctor too so that you can be prescribed medication to treat the symptoms before they grow into more serious, persistent conditions. Acquiring medial intervention is especially important when dealing with an ulcer; indeed, ulcers are extremely harmful to the lining of your organ and can be incredibly persistent if left unattended and given time to grow.

Even more, if your highly acidic diet remains the same as before the ulcer, this contributing factor will only enhance the growth of your ulcer and some of your other symptoms. Over time, the scarring of the lining within your esophagus will lead to scar tissue build up, thereby narrowing the esophagus altogether. Swallowing food and drinks will be made much more difficult as a result and may require a surgical procedure to expand the esophagus. These narrow areas of your esophagus are called strictures, and will likely lead to dangerous weight loss and or dehydration. Avoiding a procedure through immediate medical treatment of high acidity is clearly the preferred approach; but once these strictures block your esophageal pathways, a surgical procedure will be required.

Another common ailment of high acidity that affects many people is Barret's esophagus. Specifically, around 10%-15 of people who suffer from GERD will begin to also develop this painful condition, which results in dangerous changes in cells due to excess stomach acid. Thankfully, less than 1% of those who suffer from Barret's esophagus will actually develop esophageal cancer. If intervened early enough in the process, doctors are able to remove any of these abnormally developed cells through a procedure known as an endoscopy, whereby doctors will insert a flexible tube accompanied by a small camera into your esophagus. However, those who have GERD are at a, albeit slightly, increased risk of developing esophageal cancer. Even still, be sure to consult a doctor as soon as your symptoms reach a persistently painful level so that proactive measures and treatment can be implemented to quell your pain, and inhibit the growth of cancer cells.

If there is a long history of esophageal cancer in your family, you will be at an increased risk of developing this cancer as well, especially if you attain medical treatment after a prolonged period of time experiencing symptoms of high acidity. If you are aware of having a family history of esophageal cancer, make sure to ask your doctor for a regular endoscopy to find and mitigate the growth of improper cells. Moreover, tooth decay is a very common symptom of excess stomach acid as it wears down the outer layer of your teeth (enamel). As a result, this can lead to excess cavities and weakened teeth. In a recent study, researchers found that over 40% of GERD patients showed significant tooth decay, along with 70% of patients whose reflux had managed to reach the upper esophagus), compared to only 10% of those patients that had no symptoms of reflux. Certainly, reading about the symptoms that accompany stomach acid is disconcerting and worrisome. Nonetheless, being aware of the symptoms and knowing the early signs of their emergence will mitigate the risks of cancer and other chronic ailments like GERD and Barret's esophagus.

So, what can you do about these symptoms and potentially life-altering health concerns if you are experiencing excess stomach acid? Initially, and rather obviously, begin by assessing your diet. If you typically consume large meals, cut down your portions by at least 25%, and avoid eating right before you sleep. The latter is especially important for your digestive track as your body has to work harder to digest food whilst you are asleep and when your body's organs are supposed to be at rest. Also, limit your chocolate and coffee intake. Typically, medical professionals recommend limiting your coffee intake to only 2-3 cups per day at the most. If these levels are exceeded, your body's acidity levels will climb to healthy proportions and heighten your likelihood of acquiring the aforementioned symptoms. In the same way, excess consumption of alcohol and peppermint carry very harmful side-effects. Not mention, smoking is by far the most dangerous to many of your body's organs, especially the esophagus. Taking steps to cut back and eventually quit smoking is strongly recommended to not only avoid esophageal cancer and weakened tooth enamel, but for a bevy of other health-related reasons not directly associated with stomach acidity. When consulting a doctor to address stomach acid symptoms, you will most likely be prescribed an antacid, H2 blocker or a proton pump inhibitor (PPI); all three are available by prescription as well as over the counter.

Where GERD is concerned, there are other major factors that you should look out for. These symptoms are not specific to a particular body type or even certain foods. First, heartburn is, as mentioned, a clear indicator of GERD and is usually an only an occasional issue that is known to affect over 60 million people at least once or twice a month on average. However, for the 20 million individuals who suffer from heartburn on a chronic level through GERD, seemingly unrelated symptoms can inevitably result in numerous other health complications. You are well advised to consult a doctor if you find that you suffer frequent heartburn (two-three times per week regularly).

When you suffer from GERD, acid, food, as well as digestive juices tend to flow back into your esophagus from the pit of your stomach. Over time, this results in esophagitis, thereby leaving the king of the walls of the esophagus extremely vulnerable to additional harm through scarring, tearing and even deterioration. Additionally, while the primary symptom of GERD is heartburn, there are likely to be other symptoms that are far more difficult to diagnose for doctors and patients alike. Notably, doctors refer to a symptom known as, "silent reflux," which includes voice changes, chronic coughing, major and prolonged throat soreness, along with hoarseness. Patients may have a sustained sensation of having a lump in their throatier having the constant urge for having to clear one's throat. Another common symptom of GERD is the effect that stomach acid has on your breathing. Indeed, GERD, for instance, can heighten the extreme effects of asthma and or pneumonia. Whether or not patients have a history of lung problems personally or with regard to their family lineage, GERD can cause difficulty in breathing and persistent shortness of breath. However, treating this particular symptom is especially tricky; according to several recent studies, GERD medication, like PPIs, have been shown to increase pneumonia by directly contributing to the growth of harmful bacteria. Also, researchers have found that many prescribed PPIs suppress coughing that is needed to clear the lungs. As a result, your doctor may be forced to consider the function of your lungs when prescribing PPIs when in the process of treating symptoms associated with acid reflux.

Many people with ulcers from acid reflux tend to spit up blood and or see it in their stool. For a point of clarity, be sure to note that Esophageal ulcers are much different than stomach ulcers as they (stomach) are usually due to bacteria. Blood from esophageal ulcers, however, tend to be red or a darker purple-red color. If you find yourself having such symptoms, be sure to contact your doctor immediately. The immediate response from your doctor will likely be a schedules endoscopy mentioned earlier. In addition, you may also be prescribed acid-blocking or acid-reducing meds can treat these dangerous stomach ulcer.

An overarching common symptom of acid reflux is a lower quality of life. According to a 2004 study from Europe, whereby 6,000 GERD patients reported that their quality of life had been significantly diminished due to problems that are associated with drink, food and sleep, along with social and physical limitations. Not to mention, there can be major financial implications from having to buy an abundant amount of medications to treat the myriad symptoms of acid reflux, as well as the possible surgical procedures and endoscopy sessions that may be needed if the symptoms escalate to advanced stages. Moreover, the quality of life for patients of GERD was strikingly similar to heart-attack patients and was even lower, in certain cases, for those patients struggling with diabetes and cancer.

Generally, the healing time-frame for GERD is around 2 to 8 weeks. If allowed to persist without medicinal intervention, symptoms of GERD can inflict a considerable amount of damage. For example, reflux esophagitis (RO) can create visible and painful cracks and breaks in the esophageal mucosa. In order to fully and effectively heal RO, acid suppression for a prolonged period (roughly 3-9 weeks) is required and will likely be the timeframe advised by your doctor. Keep in mind that healing rates will rapidly improve as acid suppression increases.

Chronic stress is also a significant factor in the development, growth and. persistence of acid reflux. Our digestive system, moreover, is intricately associated with our nervous system. When stress presents itself, especially in an overwhelming or uncontrollable manner, our digestive system will then receive a lower amount of blood flow, thus causing various issues. Further, our gut bacteria are implicated in our management of stress at increasing levels, so probiotics are helpful in helping the management of this development.

Chapter 2: The role of Fibre, Prebiotics and Probiotics

Incorporating key changes into your diet can carry massive benefits with regard to dealing with the many symptoms of acid reflux. Specifically, consuming more fiber is an excellent way to mitigate the harsh symptoms. An important point of clarity is the distinction between dietary fiber, defined as edible but non-digestible carbohydrate-based material, and insoluble fiber. Dietary fiber is mainly available in abundance naturally in many cereals, grains, plants, and vegetables as these all play a major role in gastrointestinal health. Given the importance of fiber, and its positive impact in easing the symptoms of acid reflux, many people on average are dangerously deficient in fiber. This deficiency includes both the soluble and insoluble forms of fiber. The main difference between these two forms of fiber are found in their role in digestion; insoluble fiber expedites the travel of foods through the gastrointestinal tract, while solute fibers have been shown to slow the digestion process.

While the varied and, at times, monotonous science concerning acid reflux is still in progress and remains to be settled. Nevertheless, the theoretical benefits of adequate intake of fiber include avoiding trigger foods altogether, as well as the stomach-filling "full" effect of fiber and fewer relaxation reactions of the anti-reflux valve residing between the stomach and the esophagus. Even still, there exists a persistent relationship between acid reflux trigger and the role of fiber. To elaborate, soluble fiber has been shown to induce the body to draw fluid out of already digested food, which then contributes added bulk to your meals which leaves you with a feeling of being "full" for a far more prolonged period of time. As it is commonly found within such sources as barley, peas as well as oat bran, soluble fiber does play an active role in regulating glucose levels and may even contribute to signaling the brain that the stomach is in fact full both during and after eating a meal of any size. Moreover, smaller meals can help acid reflux by refraining from overfilling your stomach. Whereas, insoluble fiber as found within vegetables and whole grains can speed up the passage of stomach contents to your intestinal tract, thereby decreasing your body's propensity for reflux.

Additionally, fatty, fried foods are typically much lower in fiber and are also frequently accompanied by the triggering symptoms of regurgitation, indigestion, and heartburn. Indeed, a fiber-rich diet like fresh fruits, vegetables, and whole-grain bread can tend to contribute to fewer instances of reflux symptoms arising. Some dietary fibers are also widely considered to be probiotics. Note the key distinction between prebiotics and probiotics: the latter refers to the specific helpful bacteria itself, with prebiotic referring to bacterial nutrients. In other words, prebiotics are nutrients which are left for bacteria to digest, or, more plainly, fuel to encourage the balanced bacterial growth within digestive organs. Here, the role of fiber in greatly improving the many symptoms of acid reflux is illuminated; this role is as a bacterial intermediary. On the whole, nonetheless, particular items in your diet tend to perform a seemingly minor role in the symptoms associated with acid reflux. Those who suffer from chronic acid reflux are strongly advised to avoid those specific foods that can aggravate painful heartburn and regurgitation; however, eliminating a broad range of food from your diet is no recommenced as it can detrimental to your overall health. Instead, you should note foods and beverages that can trigger acid reflux specifically and root them out from your diet as soon as possible.

There is a tremendous amount of evidence in favor of incorporating a fiber-rich diet into your daily routine. Notably, the benefits are particular to the overall maintenance of your gut and with regard to managing the amount of harmful bacteria native to that region of your body. A study from 2004 that involved over 65,000 people revealed that fiber intake was associated with the improved perception of acid reflux symptoms. Also, this study revealed people who consumed high fiber bread were nearly three times as likely to experience relief of acid reflux symptoms compared to people who consumed bread with lower fiber content. Granted, the reasons for these results remains unknown; however, the authors of the broad study have speculated that the digestive process of fiber can also be a catalyst for enhanced muscle relaxation from the stomach through the esophagus as it tightens the anti-reflux valve.

So, what are the disadvantages of fiber in acid reflux? It is true that fiber is especially helpful when serving to ease acid reflux symptoms, excess fiber consumption has been shown to aggravate the symptoms. A study published in a medical journalism 2014 indicated that consuming a minimum of 10 grams of highly fermentable starches each day can significantly contribute to painful episodes of acid reflux symptoms. An additional study noted that nine participants who were diagnosed with GERD, those patients who consumed a prebiotic known as fructooligo also had elevated instances of acid reflux symptoms than those patients who were given a placebo.

There are many aspects to consider when striving to efficiently manage acid reflux symptoms. Among them, dietary fiber is perhaps the most important or, at the very least, the most consequential. For instance, while being excessively overweight is certainly risk factor as far as GERD is concerned, adequate consumption of healthy fiber will aid in keeping the weight at a healthy level. Excess fiber, however, causes stomach distension in may people, along with enhanced stomach pressure as well as prolonged emptying on the stomach in many cases, all of which have shown to lead to accentuated acid reflux symptoms. Medical professionals specializing in gastroenterology strongly recommend implementing lifestyle changes such as eating smaller sized meals on a frequent basis (as opposed to larger meals a few times per day), limiting overall consumption of carbonated beverages and foods high in salt content with the intent of improving the acid reflux symptoms. Note that women over the age of 50 should try to consume 25 grams per day; on the other hand, men under 50 are strongly advised to consume 38 grams of fiber each day. While consuming more laxatives is often the approach undertaken by people dealing with symptoms of acid reflux, medical professionals advise increasing your fiber content within your diet for maximized results, as well as maintaining your overall health as laxatives can take a substantial toll on your body and its digestive tract. Consuming a higher amount of fiber will strengthen your stool, keep wastes traveling more smoothly through your intestinal tract, along with preventing constipation. During this process of consuming more fibre, be sure to also ensure that you are consuming plenty of water as well; for fiber to have its absolute best effect, it is imperative that your body remain as hydrated as possible to make sure that waste moves smoothly along your intestinal tract rather than building up due to rigidity.

A good source of probiotics and fiber is yogurt, which carries "good" bacteria helpful for overall maintenance of gut health. A healthy gut is paramount for an efficient and well-functioning intestinal tract and digestive system. Prebiotics and probiotics are, essentially, analogous to food for the bacteria in your stomach; bananas, corn, and whole wheat are additional food sources that are high in prebiotics. Moreover, one of the most beneficial aspects of a fiber-rich diet is the notion that high-fiber foods help control your cravings for snacks. Certainly, high fiber diets can help you lose weight as it displaces other calories for overall maintenance of health.

Guarding against illness, fiber-rich diets will also lower your chances of developing major gut-related illnesses such as diverticulitis. This condition, pockets in the walls of colon trap waste as opposed to moving it along. While doctors remain unsure of the direct catalyst(s) for the illness, consuming a high-fiber diet moves waste fervently along through your system. Along with diverticulitis, a high-fiber diet also eases and prevents irritable bowel syndrome— which has also been linked to acid reflux, albeit a rarer, more extreme symptom. Nevertheless, the most common symptom of acid reflux— heartburn— is quelled by a fiber-rich diet.

Probiotics are becoming increasingly linked to the management of the symptoms associated with acid reflux and alleviating these issues. For a more technical explanation, as we are already aware that probiotics are an effective way of balancing the gut bacteria inside of our bodies, they also help combat against a bacterial infection knows as, H. pylori. This bacterial infection usually originates in childhood. This bacteria, found in the stomach, can alter the environment around them through reducing the acidity levels so that they can survive for longer periods of time. By penetrating the lining of the stomach, thereby remaining hidden and protected by the mucous membrane so that the body's immune defenses cannot reach them. In addition, these bacteria tend to secrete an enzyme called urease, which converts urea to ammonia. The presence of ammonia in this instance is significant because it reduces the stomach acidity around the specific area where the bacteria is found. Coincidentally, it is this lower stomach acid that is often mistaken— by doctors and patients alike— for acid reflux. Can probiotics help combat H. pylori? Well, many medical researchers believe that probiotics can, in fact, help battle this bacteria in several key ways. For one, probiotics are believed to strengthen the protective barrier against H. pylori by producing antimicrobial substances, along with competing against H. pylori for what is known as adhesion receptors (space on the lining of the stomach). Also, it is believed that probiotics assist in stabilizing the gut's mucosal barrier. Many researchers even argue that the production of relatively large amounts of lactate is another inhibitory factor of H. pylori due to the possibility that it could lower the H. pylori urease. Not to mention, probiotics may also be effective in modifying inflammation levels by interacting with the epithelial cells that are responsible for managing the secretion of inflammatory proteins in the gut.

Depending on the particular cause of your acid reflux, probiotics can be incredibly useful for alleviating the painful symptoms. Probiotics can be taken in conjunction with an antacid without worry of the antacid overtaking the positive benefits of the probiotic. More importantly, your approach should be to uncover the root of your acid reflux and adjust medical intervention accordingly. Of course, you doctor plays a huge role in this process, especially in diagnosing the specific cause of your acid reflux; still, it is your responsibility to seek medical expertise so that you can tackle the root of the symptoms as opposed to addressing the individual symptoms as they arise. Being aware of the triggers in both the food and drinks that you consume, managing your stress levels regardless of how often they fluctuate, and finding the specific levels of acid within your stomach are critical steps to address the symptoms of acid reflux. More likely than not, the best method of dealing with your symptoms will be to implement a diverse approach that incorporates a range of approaches rather than relying solely on medical intervention.

Chapter 3: Understanding the role of proteins, carbs, AND fats in healing acid damage

In recent years, there have been increasing reports concerning the benefits of a low-carb diet in healing the damage induced by acid damage. This may seem counterintuitive given the notion that the standard treatment for GERD includes the removal of certain foods that increase acidity in the stomach, for example, tomato sauces which are believed to be contributing causes of excess stomach acidity. Also, as mentioned in chapter 1, the removal of coffee, alcohol, smoking, and peppermint are other dietary and lifestyle changes that ease GERD symptoms. Additionally, researchers have found that diets with a higher amount of carbohydrates can significantly elevate symptoms of acid reflux. Whereas, a low-carb diet has also been shown to reduce symptoms of GERD. While many health researchers and medical experts have expressed concern over the exceptionally low proportion of daily calories from fat and protein in low-carb diets, as wells calorie levels being considerably lower in these diet than recommended. Nevertheless, the effects of gastroesophageal reflux disease have been shown to be significantly reduced after implementation of a low-carb diet. For a case in point, following a 2001 research study in which 5 individuals with diverse ranges of GERD symptoms and across the age spectrum, engaged in a low-carb diet, each of the 5 research participants showed significant relief of symptoms. Granted, throughout the duration of the study, which spanned 8 months, 3 of the 5 research participants also reduced their coffee intake concurrently.

The concurrent reduction of coffee, coupled with lower intake of carbohydrates, was shown to be effective in reducing symptoms such as heartburn and stomach pain. Interestingly, while coffee reduction was a contributing factor, observations from a few of the participants revealed that exacerbating foods such as coffee and fat are less pertinent when a low-carb diet is strictly followed. In other words, when implementing a low-carb diet, the effects of classic factors like coffee and fat intake are vastly diminished even if their consumption is not significantly reduced. So, whether or not you choose to reduce coffee and fat intake significantly, you are likely to reduce most GERD symptoms by solely undertaking a low-carb diet. Therefore, the logical conclusion to draw from these findings is that a low-carb diet is a significant factor for reducing the symptoms of acid reflux. This conclusion gains even more credibility when considering the propensity for high-carb diets to aggravate GERD symptoms.

In addition to lower carbohydrates, lean sources of protein and healthy fats are beneficial for reducing symptoms associated with acid reflux. Lean proteins found in eggs are a great addition to your diet for reducing acid reflux symptoms; however, they are a problem for many people due to elevated cholesterol. If eggs are an issue for you, be sure to consume only egg whites and refrain for consuming higher fat yolks—which have been shown to elevate GERD symptoms. Moreover, as high-fat meals and fried food typically descries LES pressure thereby delaying emptying of the stomach and boosting the risk of acid reflux, it is in your best interest to choose lean grilled meats, as well as poached, baked or broiled meats. Boosting proteins, in the way, will also provide benefits for your overall health as well. Also, complex carbohydrates, as found in rice, whole grain bread, couscous and oatmeal carry excellent benefits for reducing GERD symptoms and easing any scarring that may already be present in the walls of your esophagus. Specifically, brown rice and whole grains add valuable fiber your diet. Root vegetables such as potatoes are excellent sources of healthy carbohydrates and easily digestible fiber. Remember to refrain from incorporating too much garlic and onion while preparing your meals, which are can commonly irritate the esophagus and stomach lining.

Along with proteins and complex carbs, incorporating healthy fats has great benefits for easing GERD symptoms and other symptoms accompanying acid reflux. A type of nutrient, fat is high in calories but certainly a necessary component of your diet. Keep in mind, however, fats can vary and they do not all have the same effect on your body. On the whole, you are well advised to avoid consuming a high amount of saturated fats as typically found in dairy and meat, along with trans fats found in processed foods, shortening and margarine. As a replacement, unsaturated fats from fish and or plants are recommended; some examples of monounsaturated fats include sesame, olive, canola, sunflower, peanuts, seeds and nuts, as well as butter. In addition, examples of polyunsaturated fats include such oils as safflower, corn, flaxseed and walnut, fatty fish such as salmon and trout, along with soybean.

Some other helpful tips for reducing acid reflux symptoms include chewing gum, as long as it is not spearmint- or peppermint-flavored. Chewing gum increases the amount of saliva production in your mouth and also reduces the amount of acid in your esophagus. While alcohol consumption has already been mentioned in earlier chapters, research suggests that some people begin to experience extreme symptoms after only one drink; if you fall into this category, be sure to experiment with your levels to uncover what amount is best for you. Additionally, during and after each meal, particularly bigger meals, be sure to remain aware of your posture. Generally, it is a good idea to sit up while you are eating and avoid lying flat on your back for at least hours post-meal. Standing up and walking around the room after a big meal can help encourage the flow of gastric juices in the right direction. Further, avoiding eating big meals before bed can help you refrain from overloading your digestive system while you sleep. Digestion increases the overall amount of gastric acid that is present within your stomach. When laying down, LES's ability to inhibit stomach contents from traveling through the esophagus decreases significantly. When operating concurrently, excess stomach acid and remaining in a reclined position for an unexpended period of time create an abundance of acid reflux symptoms. On the whole, consuming a large meal for less than 3 to 4 hours prior to bed is generally not advisable for those suffering from persistent GERD symptoms; however, the timing of these symptoms can certainly vary depending on the individual.

In a 2017 research study on the benefits of healthy dietary changes versus drug intervention, researchers studied the effects of dietary changes to a type of reflux known as laryngopharyngeal reflux or LPR. This reflux is essentially triggered when pepsin, a digestive enzyme from the stomach, reaches the sensitive tissues in the upper section of the digestive tract. Symptoms like throat clearing and hoarseness are common with pepsin in the throat and or upper part of the digestive tract. In the study, the researchers had participants suffering from acid reflux switch to a Mediterranean diet and consuming significantly more water, thereby neutralizing excess acid. In this particular study, participants avoided classic triggers such as coffee, peppermint, alcohol, fatty and spicy foods, chocolate and soda. Another set of participants were given pharmaceutical drugs to ease GERD symptoms.

After a six week timeframe, participants of the study reported a greater percent of declines in their GERD symptoms as those participants that had used drugs to address the symptoms. Granted, the study did not elaborate on the particular ways in which that the diet and increased water consumption eased the symptoms; nonetheless, the Mediterranean diet incorporates eating mostly plant-based fruits and vegetables. In addition, the increased water can mitigate pepsin's acidity levels in the throat. As mentioned, fruits, vegetables and water are great methods of reducing acid reflux and GERD symptoms. With this in mind, the positive benefits experienced by the study's participants is not surprising in the least.

Adjusting your diet for GERD does not require removing all of the foods that you typically enjoy eating. Instead, a few simple changes to your diet if more than enough to address the uncomfortable symptoms of GERD. Your aim in addressing the GERD symptoms should be to create a well-rounded, nutrient-based diet that incorporates a variety of foods that include vegetables, fruits, complex carbs, healthy fats and lean sources of protein. Healing acid reflux damage is made significantly easier when starting with dietary changes that add healthy and diverse foods. Coupled with medical intervention (if required), healthy dietary changes can carry great benefits for healing scarring in your esophagus and stomach, as well as symptoms such as heartburn, bloating and even tooth decay.

Chapter 4: Exercise to reduce acid reflux

When GERD symptoms escalate and you are still in the early stages of implementing dietary changes to address acid reflux symptoms, exercise can be a great option for reducing the symptoms. When GERD symptoms begin to arise, high-impact physical activities like running, skipping rope and jumping exercises. If you are overweight or obese, a weight loss of 10% has been shown to reduce GERD symptoms like heartburn, bloating and reflux. A self-reported analysis study of individuals experiencing GERD symptoms fund that those who reduced their Body Mass Index (BMI) by 2 kilograms or 4.4 pounds or more, along with the circumference of their waist by 5cm or more has improved their GERD symptoms significantly. In contrast, there are also certain exercises that can induce reflux by opening the lower esophageal sphincter (LES) during workouts such as heavy lifting, stomach crunches, or other high impact exercises. When the LES opens, stomach acid travels up into the esophagus causing heartburn.

There are some common sense tips concerning exercise for managing GERD symptoms. First, this twice about how much and what you are eating prior to starting your exercise routine. Obviously, less food in your stomach is ideal. If you are too full, you should wait at least 1 to 2 hours before initiating your exercise routine. This will allow for food to pass fro your stomach through to the small intestine. With less food in your stomach while exercising, it is significantly less likely that you will experience the painful and annoying symptoms of acid reflux such as heartburn and bloating. Next, you should choose the food you consume with thought and, in some instances, caution. Generally, you should avoid foods that trigger GERD symptoms (choosing complex carbohydrates is advised). Your stomach does metabolize these foods much faster than others through a process known as gastric emptying. Moreover, diabetics should avoid high fat and high protein foods before exercise due to being more susceptible to experiencing slow gastric emptying. Experts also suggest adjusting your workout if you suffer from frequent GERD symptoms. Starting at a slower pace with workouts that put less strain on your body like controlled walking and controlled weight training in either a sitting or standing position is strongly recommended. Whereas, high impact, high-intensity workouts like running, rowing and cycling and induce acid reflux. Additionally, acrobatic workouts and gymnastics can also disrupt stomach contents. The key is to avoid exercises that jostle the LES and reflux, these are typically positions that put your body in awkward positions like being upside down defying gravity in one way or another.

A great exercise that carries tremendous benefits for improving and relieving acid reflux symptoms and digestion is yoga. One particular study from 2014 found that six months of yoga significantly reduced acid reflux and stomach bloating, along with improved esophagitis. Again, however, try to avoid positions that heighten GERD symptoms. If any of these "lifestyle" changes fail to improve your GERD symptoms during exercise, be sure to consult your doctor about being prescribed medication for acid-suppression. And, of course, engaging in a constant exercise routine is not only very beneficial with regard to improving your GERD symptoms, but also for the maintenance of your overall health.

Chapter 5: How to live a reflux free life?

As you may have already noticed, acid reflex can be induced by an abundance of factors ranging from diet, bad habits, poor sleep hygiene, and many other factors. Clearly, it isn't just as simple as cutting out bad habits and instilling a series of great dietary and lifestyle changes. But whether you are able to successfully implement these changes or not does not, thankfully, hinge on strict adherence to a stringent diet or eliminating some of your favorite guilty habits. But before you can begin to consider stepping into a reflux-free life, you should be cognizant of the stages of reflux and recovery.

Firstly, almost everyone who suffers from GERD begins with normal LES and little to no reflux. The severity level of GERD, therefore, more than likely correlates to best with the overall degree of damage inflicted upon the sphincter. Note, however, that this is not easy to determine. Normally, the amount of damage to your sphincter correlates with the overall severity of acid reflux symptoms. This severity is most often determined by the volume, frequency, and duration of reflux episodes. In turn, these factors will correlate with GERD symptoms such as regurgitation and heartburn. If you are diagnosed with GERD, your strategy for addressing the symptoms and eventually overcoming them should first be to containment. Unfortunately, damage to your LES caused by GERD cannot be reversed by drugs and is permanent. Nonetheless, many patients of GERD have been able to live with these symptoms and with functionality despite damage to the sphincter. Changing simple lifestyle habits, such as sleeping and eating, can significantly decrease and prevent severe reflux episodes in spite of damage to your sphincter.

In Stage 1 of GERD, known as Mild GERD, most adults currently have minimal damage to their LES and tend to experience mild GERD occasionally. Most often, the adults are left with either tolerating occasional heartburn or will have to use over-the-counter acid suppressive medications from the onset of symptoms through its subsequent stages. Typically, when taking drugs to address the symptoms, quality of life for patients is not affected because the medications are very effective in suppressing symptoms. If you choose to take medication to address symptoms, make sure that you are also cleaning up your diet. If you continue to consume trigger foods and beverages, like coffee and certain sauces, for example, the benefits you garner from medication will be minimal and your recovery will be prolonged if not inhibited altogether. Replacing these meals with smaller, leaner meals that do not pose a threat to inducing symptoms of GERD is recommended. This will ease heartburn and lessen the damage to your sphincter.

In stage 2, known as Moderate GERD, symptoms are far more difficult to control and use of prescribed acid-suppressive drugs will be needed. In this stage, reflux is accompanied by symptoms that are far more intense than stage 1. Therefore, medicinal intervention is needed to mitigate the damage and pain caused by these symptoms. Still, many symptoms in this stage can be managed by using acid-suppressive drugs for prolonged periods of time. Keep in mind that over-the-counter medication can provide insufficient relief; whereas, prescription strength medications are needed in order for you to manage GERD symptoms effectively. Additionally, stage 3, or, Severe GERD, can result in a very low quality if life and is generally considered to be an extremely serious problem by medical professionals specializing in GERD. Because prescription grade acid-suppressive drugs and medicinal intervention usually do not control symptoms, regurgitation is frequent. In Stage 3, it is entirely possible that complications associated with erosive GERD are present. Lastly, stage 4, or, reflux-induced esophageal cancer, is quite obviously the most serious stage. The result of numerous years of severe reflux, nearly 16% of all long-term reflux sufferers progress to this extremely advanced stage. Due to the long-term reflux, the esophagus' lining has been heavily damaged, thereby resulting in a high degree of cellular changes. Also, stage 4 is the stage that involves the pre-cancerous condition called Barrett's esophagus and or an even more severe condition called dysplasia. Granted, these conditions are not cancerous. However, they are capable of raising the risk of developing reflux-induced esophageal cancer. Accordingly, at this stage, common GERD symptoms are likely to also be accompanied by a strong burning sensation in the throat, chronic coughing, and persistent hoarseness. A narrowing of the esophagus, or strictures, will also be present in this stage, and can also be characterized by the sensation that food is sticking to your throat. However, this is only a feeling associated with strictures. Notably, this symptom is also caused by esophageal cancer. Keep in mind that stage 4 GERD can only be diagnosed by a medical professional through an endoscopy and from an intrusive biopsy of cells retrieved from the lower esophagus.

A 30-day recovery plan for GERD symptom can be easily broken into weekly steps. In the first week, you will presumably be trying to lean off of the medication that you have been prescribed. A reversion plan of this nature should take into account a variety of approaches that incorporate dietary changes, exercise routines, sleep schedules, and other lifestyle changes. Drinking more tea and water is strongly recommended throughout your 30-day reversion plan, as long as the tea is not peppermint-flavored. Also, in your first week of recovery, be sure to get as much sleep as possible, in conjunction with eating 2 to 3 hours before you sleep. A meal should also be incorporated throughout this entire 30-day stretch. This plan should include egg whites in the morning, instead of coffee switch to tea for your caffeine fix. For lunch, whole grain bread with lean meat- chicken or turkey preferably- with light sauce and a bevy of vegetables. Moreover, dinner should include a balanced meal that provides nutrients and foods that will not induce heartburn. Remember, this meal should be consumed a few hours before bed so that your body has time to properly digest the food. Also, be sure to refrain from lying directly on your back after your meal; as mentioned, this will induce acid reflux symptoms like heartburn and excess bloating.

In week 2, in keeping with the consumption of nutrient-rich food and water consumption from the previous week, you should begin an exercise routine of you have been devoid of routine prior to week 2. A consistent exercise routine will help maintain overall health so that your body has excess strength and energy to overcome the wear and damage inflicted from GERD symptoms. Also, a consistent exercise routine will boost your metabolism so that you can burn off excess unhealthy fats and complex carbohydrates that can cause strain to your body and induce reflux symptoms. In the third week of your 30-day revision plan, you can slightly increase the size of your meals. Still, make sure that the overall size of your meals remain relatively small, with only slight additions where you may see fit. By week three, your exercise routine, water consumption, and sleep habits should be starting to feel more routine and many of reflux your symptoms will begin to diminish. Moreover, leading into week 4, your diet should continue to incorporate nuts, vegetables, fruits, tea, and other plant-based foods and drinks to expedite the healing process. However, the final week of your 30-day recovery plan is vital for sustaining the progress that you have presumably made since the start of the month. It is vital because you must ensure that you do not get too comfortable in your routine that you allow for gradual decline back into the habits that spawned your acid reflux. Pushing through this final week will augment your progress and solidify your path to living a reflux-free life. Specifically, with regard to your diet, you can incorporate the following fruit and vegetable smoothie recipe. Smoothies and healthy shakes are an excellent meal replacement option for optimal health and recovery from acid reflux.

1. Add 2 scoops of frozen berries into a 400ml cup
2. Add 2 scoops of spinach from a 250ml scoop
3. Add 2 tablespoons of Chia Seeds
4. Add 2 tablespoons of hemp hearts
5. Add 1 tablespoon of peanut butter

This smoothie should be blended with water to ensure that it is not excessively thick.

PART 2

Chapter 1: What in the world is a thyroid

In this chapter, we will be exploring just what the thyroid is, and its functions in maintaining and keeping your body healthy.

For starters, the word thyroid has its origins dating as far back as the 1690s. Coming from the Greek, thyreoiedes, meaning "shield-shaped". Also referred to as, khondros thyreoiedes, "shield-shaped cartilage". Aptly named, as the thyroid gland is an organ which is often considered to resemble a butterfly, bow tie, or shield shape, at the base of the neck.

The thyroid gland plays an extremely vital role in the way your body uses energy, by releasing hormones that aid in controlling your body's metabolism. The hormones released by the thyroid gland assist in regulating important body functions, including but not limited to:

- Regulation of breathing
- Heart rate
- The central and peripheral nervous systems
- Body weight
- Cycles of menstruation
- The strength of muscles
- Levels of cholesterol
- The temperature of the body

Quite a lot for an organ coming in at only around 2 inches long. This tiny but important gland rests in the front portion of the throat, in front of the trachea, and just below the thyroid cartilage commonly referred to as the

Adam's apple. The Adam's apple itself is the largest cartilage of the voice box or larynx.

Owing to the bow tie, butterfly, or shield shape, of the thyroid gland, is a middle connection of thin thyroid tissue, which is known as the isthmus, which is responsible for holding together two lobes on the right and left sides of it. It is not entirely uncommon, however, for someone to be missing the isthmus all-together and instead of having the two lobes of the thyroid gland operating separate from one another.

Now that you are aware of this and may feel a bit more familiar with your own thyroid gland, you may resist trying to see or feel around for it in your neck yourself. Unless the thyroid gland is otherwise afflicted and made to become enlarged, mostly known as a goiter, the thyroid will be unable to be seen, and only just barely able to be felt. It is only when a goiter occurs and the neck is swollen from an enlarged thyroid that it will be at all noticeable either to the eye or to the touch.

The thyroid gland is one of the major players in the endocrine system. The endocrine system includes glands that are responsible for the production and for the secretion of various hormones. The other organs which help make up the endocrine system are the hypothalamus, which is responsible for linking the body's nervous system to the endocrine system via the use of the pituitary gland. The pituitary gland which is responsible for the secretion of hormones, not the blood stream. The pineal gland, which produces the wake/sleep pattern hormone of melatonin. The adrenal glands, which are responsible for the production of a variety of hormones like the steroids cortisol and aldosterone as well as our body's adrenaline.

The Pancreas, an organ located in the abdominal region of the body, the primary role of which is the converting of food into fuel for the body's cells. The ovaries and testicles, sex organs of the body. And the parathyroid glands.

Utilizing the iodine content from foods, the thyroid is able to produce and churn out the hormones T3, which stands for triiodothyronine, and the hormone T4, thyroxine.

T3, or triiodothyronine, is merely the active form of the companion hormone thyroxine, or T4. The thyroid gland alone is able to secrete around 20% of our body's T3 into the bloodstream on its own. With the other 80% coming from organs like the liver and the kidneys going through the process of converting thyroxine into its active counterpart.

It is absolutely possible for your body to have far too much of T3 though. When there is an over secretion of T3 into the blood stream, it is called thyrotoxicosis. This can be due to a number of conditions dealing with the thyroid gland such as overactivity in the thyroid gland, known as hyperthyroidism, caused by such conditions as a benign tumor, the thyroid gland becoming enflamed, or a condition known as graves' disease. The previously mentioned condition of a goiter, in which the neck begins to swell, might be a signal of thyrotoxicosis having occurred. Even more symptoms to have an eye out for in case of hyperthyroidism will be an increase in the appetite, increased regularity of bowel movements, an intolerance to heat, the loss of weight, the menstrual cycle becoming irregulated, a heartbeat becoming increasingly rapid or irregular in rhythm, the thinning or loss of hair, tremors, becoming irritable, overly tired, palpitations, and the eyelids retracting.

It is also possible for your body to be producing too little of the hormone T3. The thyroid gland producing too little of T3 is known commonly as hypothyroidism. It is common for autoimmune diseases to have a strong role in this occurring, an example of which would be the Hashimoto's disease, which causes the immune system to attack the thyroid gland. Certain medications or the intake of too little iodine can also cause hypothyroidism. This can be very serious, especially if a case of hypothyroidism goes unnoticed or untreated during early childhood, or even before birth. With the regulation of hormones being so important, primarily to physical and mental development, not treating hypothyroidism during these crucial times often result in reduced growth for the child, or becoming learning disabled.

The affliction of hypothyroidism is not foreign to adults though. When hypothyroidism occurs in adults they tend to have the functions of their bodies slowed down drastically. The effects of hypothyroidism in an adult have been known to include symptoms such as a growing intolerance to colder temperature, the heart rate of the adult will lower, gaining weight, a reduction in appetite, the ability of memory becomes poorer, fertility will reduce, muscles will become stiff, the adult may become depressed, and tired.

T4, or thyroxine, is the primary hormone that gets secreted from the thyroid gland and into the body's bloodstream. Unlike T3 which is active, thyroxine is in an inactive form and most of it will need to be converted to the active form, triiodothyronine, which is a process that takes place in organs like the kidneys and liver. Undergoing these processes is vital in making sure the body is able to regulate a healthy metabolic rate, control of the body's muscles, development of the brain, develop and maintain bones, and digestive and heart functionality.

As with T3, triiodothyronine, the production and secretion of too much will inevitable result in thyrotoxicosis, while the production and secretion of too little thyroxine, will result in hypothyroidism.

To combat this, the body and thyroid gland have a few tricks vital to the regulation of levels of these hormones in the cells. There is a controlled feedback loop system, involving the hypothalamus in the brain as well as in the thyroid gland and pituitary gland which is in control of the production of both of the hormones thyroxine and triiodothyronine. Thyrotropin-releasing hormones are secreted from the hypothalamus and, in turn, the pituitary gland becomes stimulated into producing thyroid stimulating hormone. A hormone which will stimulate thyroxine and triiodothyronine to be produced and secreted by the thyroid gland.

A feedback loop regulates this production system, to account for the levels of thyroxine and of triiodothyronine. If the levels of either of these thyroid gland hormones begin to increase, they will end up preventing the production and secretion of the thyrotropin-releasing hormone as well as the thyroid stimulating hormone, thus allowing the body to maintain, on it's own, a steady level of the thyroid hormones that it needs.

For all these reasons it is of vital importance that the levels of T3 and T4 being secreted thru-ought the body and its cells never get too high or too low. T3 and T4 are able to reach just about ever cell in the body by utilizing the bloodstream. The rate of work for the cells and metabolism to work is regulated by the hormones T3 and T4. To make sure that levels are never either too high or too low, this is why we have a thyroid gland.

The final hormone that the thyroid gland is responsible for the production of is the hormone calcitonin, CT, or thyrocalcitonin. Within the thyroid gland are what are known as C-cells, or parafollicular cells, which are in charge of the proliferation of this particular hormone. The primary role of calcitonin in the body is to help in the regulation of the levels of phosphate in the blood, and of calcium in the blood. Doing so is to be in opposition of the parathyroid hormone. In short, meaning that what it aims to do is reduce the amount of calcium in the blood stream. The reason for playing this role in the human anatomy game has been a bit of a mystery to science up to this point though, due to the observation of patients showing either very high or even very low levels of the hormone calcitonin, having no adverse effect on them.

The hormone calcitonin has two primary mechanisms by which to aid in the reduction of calcium levels within the human body. It can completely inhibit the activity of the cells in our body which are responsible for breaking down bones, known as osteoclasts. Osteoclasts do this because when bone is broken down, the calcium within the bone being broken down will be released into the body's bloodstream. So by inhibiting the osteoclasts from doing their respective jobs, calcitonin is directly involved in the reduction of the amount of calcium that is getting released into the body's bloodstream. Despite doing this though, the length of time that calcitonin can cause this inhibition has been shown to be quite short. Calcitonin can be an active player in the resorption of calcium into the kidneys, which it does by lower the levels of blood calcium in the body.

Calcitonin has been manufactured in the past and has then been given, in this form, to treat the disease of bone, Paget's disease. Also known as osteitis deformans, Paget's disease is rather common, and is a chronic bone disorder which can cause pain, fractures or deformities of a bone, or show absolutely no symptoms at all. It is however easily able to be controlled and treated with proper early enough diagnosis and treatment.

The manufactured hormone calcitonin has also been given to sufferers of general bone pain, and of hypercalcaemia, which is when the body has an abnormal level of calcium flowing in the bloodstream.

Though because of the introduction of bisphosphonates, which aid in the preventing of the breakdown of bone cells and are drugs also used to help treat osteoporosis, the use of manufactured calcitonin has decreased.

Chapter 2: possible thyroid disorders

In the previous chapter, we began to cover what it is exactly that the thyroid gland gets done and even dabbled a bit into how it does it's job properly. During the last chapter, we mentioned a few of the various thigs which can afflict the thyroid gland, why this may occur in certain circumstances, and what the effects of these afflictions could be. Moving on into chapter two is where we will begin to take a closer look at everything that can go wrong with the thyroid gland. Not just the what, but the why as well. What causes these changes in our thyroid gland to occur, and what to expect to happen when they do occur. The importance of having this knowledge be a part of your thyroid gland arsenal cannot be at all overstated as there is a wide array of severity to both the symptoms and to the results of the ailments that can afflict the thyroid gland and consequently hinder our body's ability to maintain its health properly.

Just as well in this chapter, you can expect to be reading deeper into some of the ailments that may have already been brought up in the previous chapter, such as hyperthyroidism, hypothyroidism, graves disease, goiters, and Hashimoto's disease.

Hyperthyroidism

As briefly discussed in the last chapter, hyperthyroidism is a rather common condition in which there is overactivity in the thyroid gland and begins to produce far too much of the thyroid hormone which would usually be used to regulate the body's metabolic rate. This can be an overproduction of the hormones T3, which is triiodothyronine, T4, which is tetraiodothyronine, or even an overproduction of both of these hormones.

The causes of hyperthyroidism can vary greatly, with the most common reason for it being the aforementioned Grave's disease, which we will go much further into later in the chapter. The basics of Grave's disease are that it is an autoimmune disorder which causes antibodies in the body to stimulate the thyroid gland making it secrete to many of it's hormones. You should tell your regular doctor if any one in your family has ever had Grave's disease as it seems to have a genetic link, being passed down commonly from generation to the next generation. Grave's disease is also known to be more prevalent in women, affecting about 1 percent of the female population, than it is in men.

Another common reason for hyperthyroidism to occur is an excess level of iodine in the body, which is the main ingredient in hormones T3 and T4.

Less common, but still just as relevant to the conversation as causes for hyperthyroidism is thyroiditis which is the inflammation of thyroid gland, which in turn will cause the hormones T3 and T4 to start leaking out of the thyroid gland.

Tumors located on the ovaries or testes have been known links to hyperthyroidism. As well as even tumors, even when benign, located on the thyroid gland, or pituitary gland.

An easily preventable cause of hyperthyroidism which should not be overlooked is the intake of large amounts of T4, or tetraiodothyronine, via the ingestion of a dietary supplement or of a prescribed medication.

When it comes to the symptoms of hyperthyroidism, believe it or not, we had only scratched the surface in the previous chapter and will be going more in-depth here on what you can expect to look out for in order to self-diagnose an issue before going to seek out a professional opinion.

To begin with, in the case of Grave's disease, one of the symptoms can be a bulging of the eyes as if stuck in a stare. Other symptoms to watch out for would be an increase in the appetite, perhaps an increase in nervousness or a sense of restlessness. Muscular weakness, the inability to concentrate on simple tasks, irregularity in the heartbeat, loss of the ability to sleep soundly or for long periods of time, the loss of hair, or noticing that your hair has become thinner or more brittle, can be signs of hyperthyroidism. Thinness of the skin is also common, as well as becoming more irritable, sweating more, or becoming more anxious. In men specifically, the development of breasts can be a sign of hyperthyroidism. And in women, hyperthyroidism has been known to have adverse effects on the regularity of the menstrual cycle.

If you experience any of the prior symptoms, it is, of course, recommended to seek out professional help and diagnosis. However, it is highly recommended that you seek out professional help for the treatment of hyperthyroidism if you begin to experience a sensation of dizziness if you start to notice shortness in your breathing, which will likely come with the increase in heart rate, making it faster and irregular, and any loss of consciousness. Having hyperthyroidism has also been known to be the cause of atrial fibrillations, which are a dangerous arrythmia, commonly responsible for leading to having a stroke, or even to congestive heart failures.

In diagnosing a case of hyperthyroidism, a doctor will likely begin the process by conducting a full and complete medical history, as well as a physical exam. These are commonly conducted as they are helpful in revealing the common signs of loss of weight, how rapid your pulse is, an elevation in pressure of the blood, protrusion of the eyes, or the enlargement of the thyroid gland itself.

It is also reasonable to expect your doctor to conduct a cholesterol test which will be done to check on the levels of cholesterol in your system. This is done because cholesterol levels being low can be an indication that there is an elevation in your metabolic rate, which would mean that your body is burning through your cholesterol far too quickly.

Doctors are also able to conduct tests to measure the levels of T3 and T4 that are in your blood. Thyroid stimulating hormone tests can be done to check the levels of TSH, or thyroid stimulating hormone coursing within your body. TSH stimulates your thyroid gland to produce the hormones the body needs, and if your thyroid gland is producing levels of hormones at a normal rate, or even a rate that is too high, your TSH should come out lower. And a level of TSH that is abnormally low can be an important signifier that you may have hyperthyroidism.

A triglyceride test will be done, because similarly to having low amounts of cholesterol, a low level of triglycerides can be significant of an elevation in your metabolic rate. A thyroid scan or uptake will allow a doctor to see if your thyroid gland is being overactive. It will actually get even more particular, and let a doctor be able to see if it is the entire thyroid gland which is acting up or just a particular area of the thyroid gland.

Ultrasounds have been known to be utilized, as they will allow a doctor to observe entirely, the size of the thyroid gland, as well as any masses that may be within the thyroid gland. It is the use of the ultrasound which will also be able to let the doctor know if the mass inside the thyroid gland is cystic, or if it is solid. Just as well a CT, Computed Tomography, or MRI, Magnetic Resonance Imaging, scan can be performed to show if the condition is being caused by a tumor being present on the pituitary gland.

Treatment of hyperthyroidism also comes in varieties and may be dependent on the cause of the hyperthyroidism. Perhaps the most common treatment comes in the form of medication. Generally an antithyroid medication like methimazole, also known as Tapazole, which will cause the thyroid gland to halt the production and secretion of hormones altogether.

According to the American Thyroid Association, around 70 percent of U.S. adults who undergo treatment for hyperthyroidism will receive a form of treatment called radioactive iodine. Radioactive iodine is essentially able to completely and effectively destroy the cells that would otherwise be producing hormones. Radioactive iodine, or RAI, in the form of a liquid or a pill, will be ingested by way of the mouth, and is safe to use on an individual who has had any allergic reaction to an X-ray contrast agent or to seafood, because essentially the reaction comes from the compound which contains iodine, and not from the iodine itself. The iodine, in an iodide form, is actually split into two forms or radioactive iodine, known as I-123, which is harmless to thyroid gland cells, and I-131, which is responsible for the destruction of thyroid gland cells. The radiation which is emitted by both of these forms of the iodine are able to be detected from outside of the patient, which will help the doctor to gain any information needed the thyroid glands functionality, and take any pictures needed of the size thyroid glands tissues, as well as their location in the body. This treatment is not without its side effects though, which generally tend to come in the presence of dryness of the mouth, soreness of the eyes and in the throat, and has also been known to effect changes in taste. You may also be required, if undergoing this treatment, to take precautions for a short time which will prevent the spread of radiation to others.

Surgery is yet another common form of treatment for hyperthyroidism. In this case, it is entirely possible that a section of your thyroid gland will be removed, though entire thyroid glands have also been removed in this procedure. This is followed up with taking thyroid hormone supplements which will help in the prevention of hypothyroidism, which is what happens when there is the occurrence of underactivity in the thyroid gland, causing it to produce and secrete too little of the intended hormones. Beta-blockers may also be taken, such as something like propranolol to help control a rapid pulse, sweating, any anxiety that may crop up, and higher blood pressure. It is reported that most people respond very well to this form of treatment.

If you would like to improve any symptoms, or even take action to prevent symptoms from occurring, you are not left without options. You can work along with your doctor, or a dietician, to help create a healthy guideline for diet, exercise, and any nutritional supplementation. Proper diet intake, with a stronger focus on getting calcium and sodium, can be crucially important in the prevention of hyperthyroidism. Osteoporosis is a common result of hyperthyroidism as it can make your bones become thin, weak, and very brittle. To strengthen the bones after treatment for hyperthyroidism, it is recommended to take calcium supplements and vitamin D. To get an idea of how much vitamin D you should be taking post-surgery, you can talk to your doctor for a recommendation.

Moving on from treatment, it is not unusual for a doctor to recommend their patients to an endocrinologist, who will be more specialized in the treatment of systems dealing with bodily hormones. You'll want to avoid stress at this stage as it can cause thyroid storm, which happens when a large amount of thyroid hormone gets released, resulting in a horrible and sudden worsening of any prior symptoms. Proper treatment is both recommended and effective at the prevention of thyroid storm, as well as other complications such as thyrotoxicosis.

In the long-term, the outlook for something like hyperthyroidism is dependent heavily on what is causing it. Some of the causes of hyperthyroidism can go away without ever seeking treatment. Whereas a more serious cause like Graves' disease is not to be taken lightly, as it will get much worse if it goes without treatment, and the complications due to Graves' disease are often life-threatening and will have an affect on your quality of life long-term. These are easy enough to subdue with proper care and an early diagnosis and treatment.

Hypothyroidism

Though we went over a little about hypothyroidism in chapter 1, it is important to take a closer look at the disorder, to gain a better idea of its symptoms, and proper treatment and care for it.

When the body is not producing enough of the thyroid hormones that it needs, this is what is known as hypothyroidism having occurred. This will cause the general functions of your body to become slowed down, as the thyroid gland is responsible for producing and secreting hormones which will provide energy to nearly every other portion of your body. Though this affliction can come to task at any age, it is more common for an underactive thyroid gland to be noticed in adults over the age of 60, as well as being more prevalent in women. A diagnosis of hypothyroidism is nothing to get too worked up about, fortunately, as treatment of hypothyroidism has been known to be quite effective, as well as being very simple and very safe.

Though the symptoms of having an underactive thyroid gland can vary from person to person, there is enough overlap in the symptoms for us to help lay out what to look out for. It is important to note, however, that there can be difficulty in pin-pointing that a symptom is that of hypothyroidism and that the severity of the condition itself plays a large role in which signs or symptoms will appear, as well as when they may make an appearance.

It is not at all uncommon for most people to experience the symptoms of this condition arriving in a slow progression over many years. The thyroid gland will grow ever slower and slower, which will only then allow the symptoms to be better identifiable. The trouble can become that many of the symptoms come with general aging, so if you suspect there is more to the picture, and that hypothyroidism is at play, it is important to go see a doctor. An example of some early symptoms which also come naturally with age are the symptomatic fatigue and gaining of weight.

If hypothyroidism does occur, however, other symptoms to keep an eye out for will be an uptick in depression, constipation, or muscle weakness. It is also common to begin becoming more sensitive to the cold, for the skin to become dry, and a reduction in sweating. Your heart rate will generally become slower, blood cholesterol may elevate, and joints may become stiff or experience more pain. It is also possible for memory to start becoming impaired, hair may thin or become dry. Your voice may become hoarse, muscles will stiffen and experience soreness, your face will become puffy and sensitive. In women, hypothyroidism as been known to negatively affect menstrual changes and cause difficulty in fertility.

When it comes to the causes of hypothyroidism, an autoimmune disease is fairly common to be the culprit at work. The body is designed in such a way that your immune system generally will protect the body's cells against any invading bacteria and virus. Therefore, when an unknown virus or bacteria enters the body, it is the immune system which will respond by sending out what are known as fighter cells, to destroy the foreign invading virus or bacteria.

However, it is not impossible for your body to begin confusing what are the healthy and normal cells, with the invading cells. This is what is then called an autoimmune response to the cells. And if this autoimmune response does not get properly treated, or if it is not properly regulated, it is your own immune system which will start to attack your healthy body tissues. Medically, this has been known to cause quite serious issues, which include hypothyroidism.

Hashimoto's disease, which we have mentioned before, is one such autoimmune condition that can occur, and it is the most common among the causes of having an underactive thyroid gland. The disease literally will attack the thyroid gland which will cause chronic thyroid inflammation, which, in turn, will reduce the functionality of the thyroid gland. As with Graves' disorder having links between generations, it is not at all uncommon to find that multiple members of a family have this same condition as well.

Hypothyroidism can even become an occurrence as a result of treatment for hyperthyroidism, which has the aim of lowering your thyroid hormone. It is not uncommon for the treatment to result in keeping the thyroid hormone too low, which then becomes hypothyroidism, which has been a known result of the radioactive iodine treatment for hyperthyroidism.

The surgical removal of the thyroid gland is yet another known cause of the occurrence of hypothyroidism. The entirety of the thyroid gland will be removed in the case of thyroid problems cropping up, which will affect the body's ability to produce thyroid hormone, and cause hypothyroidism. In this instance, you will typically be recommended to take thyroid medication for the rest of your life. In the case that it is only a smaller portion of the thyroid gland which is removed, it is possible for the thyroid gland to still be able to produce and secrete a healthy amount of hormones. In which case it will take a test of the blood to determine how much medication you will need.

It is possible for radiation therapy to be the cause if you have come down with hypothyroidism. A diagnosis of leukemia, neck cancer, or lymphoma will likely mean you have had to undergo a form of radiation therapy, which very nearly almost leads to the occurrence of hypothyroidism.

Just as possible, is a medication you may be taking to lower thyroid gland hormone production, to be the cause of hypothyroidism. Medications such as these are commonly used in the treatment of certain psychological diseases, and even have been known to be used in treating heart disease and cancer.

When it comes down the diagnosing of hypothyroidism, there are two primary methods which have been favored and work to best identify when it has occurred. The first being a strict medical evaluation, much like in the case of checking for hyperthyroidism. The doctor will give you a very thorough exam physically, as well as making sure to go over your medical history. Hypothyroidism has a couple physical signs which the doctor will be checking for primarily such as the dryness of the skin, how slow or quick your reflexes are, any swelling of the neck, and the rate of your heart beat. It is at this time that a doctor will also likely ask you to report any of the other symptoms listed earlier that you may have experienced, such as the depression, any fatigue, if you have been constipated, and a sensation of being more sensitive to the cold. It is also at this point it will be most helpful for you to let the doctor know of any thyroid conditions which have existed in your family.

To reliably get an idea of the existence of hypothyroidism in the body, it is required to conduct blood tests. It is only by this method that anyone will be able to tell and get a look at a measure of your body's thyroid-stimulating hormone levels, done by utilizing a thyroid-stimulating hormone test to see how much of the thyroid-stimulating hormone your pituitary gland is or is not creating. In the case that your thyroid gland is not producing enough of the hormone, the pituitary gland will respond to this by boosting the thyroid-stimulating hormone it produces in order to increase thyroid hormone production. If it turns out you have hypothyroidism, the levels of thyroid-stimulating hormone in your body will be increased, because your body is responding by making an attempt at stimulating more thyroid gland hormone activity. If hyperthyroidism is what ails you, the levels of the thyroid-stimulating hormone in your body will as having decreased, because in this case, your body has begun the process of attempting to halt the function of excessive production of the thyroid glands hormones.

Another useful method in the detection and diagnosis of hypothyroidism is to test the levels of T4 in the body, being produced by your thyroid gland, as T4 is produced directly by the thyroid gland. When they are used in conjunction with one another, a test of T4 levels and the thyroid-stimulating hormone test are very helpful in coming up with an evaluation of thyroid gland functionality. In general, if you the levels of thyroid-stimulating hormone in your body has increased, while the level of the hormone T4 has decreased, you much more than likely have hypothyroidism. Though, due to the sheer amount of conditions that can have such a negative impact on the thyroid gland, it could very well end up being necessary to conduct even more tests of the thyroid glands function

I order to properly diagnose the issue.

Though it is true that for many people who have thyroid conditions, that the right amount of the proper medication will assist in the alleviation of their symptoms, you will have hypothyroidism for the rest of your life if you get it.

To get the best of hypothyroidism it is most commonly treated the best with the use of levothyroxine, also known as Levothroid or Levoxyl, which is T4 put into a synthetic form that is responsible for copying the action the thyroid hormone would regularly take if it were being produced as normal by your body. The idea behind doing this is that the medication will cause a return to the proper levels of the thyroid hormone in your blood. Once a restoration of the thyroid hormone level has occurred, many of the symptoms that come along with having hypothyroidism, will at the very least become much easier to manage, and at best the hypothyroidism symptoms will disappear altogether. It is important to expect it to take several weeks, following treatment, before relief sets in, and you start to feel a return to normalcy. There will also very likely be follow up appointments for testing your blood, which the doctor will recommend in order to keep a solid eye on your progress into recovery. Chances are that you will also receive some medication or other recommended methods to aid you in your recovery, be sure to speak with your doctor about the dosage you should be taking and to come up with a solid plan, that will most benefit you, for recovering in a timely fashion.

It is the case that many people who end up with hypothyroidism medicate for it, for the rest of their lives. Despite this, the dosage you will be taking thru ought that time is likely to go through changes. To better get an idea of how these dosages should be changing over time, it is best to get a check up on your thyroid-stimulation hormone levels every year. In this way, your doctor will be able to more properly adjust the amount you should be taking, or not taking, based on the blood levels indicated by the thyroid-stimulating hormone tests. Only by doing this regularly, will you and your doctor be able to achieve the recovery program that works best for you.

Plans and programs for this achievement may include medications and other hormone supplementation. Once again, synthetic versions of the hormone you need may be used, as they are a widely used and viable practice to aid in the recovery of hypothyroidism. The synthetic version of the hormone T3 is liothyronine, and T4 in its synthetic medication form is called levothyroxine, both of which act as suitable substitutes for their corresponding hormone.

If it was a deficiency in your iodine intake which caused your specific occurrence of hypothyroidism, it is likely that your doctor will recommend a supplementary form of iodine. Keep in mind to ask your doctor, and get the proper testing before taking anything, but selenium and magnesium supplements have been known to aid heavily in the treatment of hypothyroidism.

The golden ticket to any recovery or treatment is usually diet, and in the case of hypothyroidism, there is no exception. Though this is the case, and diet can be incredibly beneficial in your recovery and treatment, do not expect a change in your diet, doctor recommended or otherwise, to replace the need for a prescribed medication. Foods that are rich in selenium or magnesium such as nuts and seeds like the Brazil nut and sunflower seeds have been shown to be very beneficial additions to any diet to aid in the treatment of hypothyroidism.

Balance in your diet will play an especially important role, as the thyroid gland requires particular amounts of iodine in order to properly reach full functionality. There are foods such as whole grains, vegetables, fruits, and lean meats which can handily accomplish this without the need for iodine supplementation.

And of course, diet is only the beginning, exercise as well comes in as an important slice of the treatment and recovery pie. The muscle and joint pain that coincides with hypothyroidism will more often than not leave one to feel extreme fatigue and depression, both of which can be helped by creating and sticking to a regular work out regime. Though no exercise should be discounted, unless specifically told to avoid certain activities by your doctor, there are certain ones which will prove more beneficial than others for treating the symptoms of hypothyroidism. Low impact workouts such as swimming, riding a bike, doing Pilates or yoga, or even a good brisk walk, have been known to be very helpful low impact work outs that are helpful and easy to work in to a daily routine.

The building up of muscle mass by strength training, lifting weights, sit ups, pushups, and pull-ups, help reduce the lethargic feeling of sluggishness that comes along with hypothyroidism. The increase in muscle mass will result in an increase in the rate of your metabolism, which will simultaneously assist in decreasing any weight gain that the hypothyroidism may have caused.

And finally doing training that is primarily cardiovascular. As stated earlier, hypothyroidism is one of the ailments that can correlate with a heightened risk of having a cardiac arrythmia, or irregularity of the heartbeat. By taking steps to be more mindful of your cardiovascular health, exercising on a regular basis or schedule, will help in protecting your heart.

There are also alternative treatments which exist to help in taking care of hypothyroidism, such as animal extracts that contain the thyroid hormone. These extracts are made available from pigs because they contain both the thyroid hormone T4 and thyroid hormone T3. It is uncommon for these to be recommended, however, as they have not shown to be reliable in how to dose, as well as not being more effective than the typically recommended medications. It is also popular to find some glandular extracts in stores that are health food based. The risk that comes along with them is that the U.S. Food and Drug Administration plays no role in the monitoring or the regulation of these extracts. This has historically brought the guarantee of their pureness, legitimacy, and even their potency into question. If you decide to use these products, you do so at your own risk, but still be sure to inform your doctor so that they can adjust accordingly to your treatment.

You can go above and beyond in regards to hypothyroidism treatment, yet still deal with issues or complications that are longer lasting because of this harsh fluctuation to your body. Luckily there have been methods developed and used which will help to lessen the burden of hypothyroidisms effects on your life moving forward.

In the beginning, fatigue can feel like a lot to deal with, especially when associated with depression. These feelings can creep through even if you are taking proper dosages of your medication. It is of utmost importance that you get a good quality sleep every night to ease your treatment and recovery. A good, healthy diet, as well as the relief of stress through activities such as meditation, Pilates, and yoga, are effective strategies when it comes to combating lower energy levels.

It is also vitally important to recognize the difficulty of having a medical condition that is chronic, especially in the case of something like hypothyroidism, which comes along with its own mixed bag of other concerns to your overall health. Being able to talk about, or express, the experience of going through this will help. There are resources out there for support groups of other people who live with the effects of hypothyroidism, you can find a therapist to talk to, perhaps a close friend or loved one. Anyone who will be able to enable you to discuss your experience with openness and with honesty. You may even be able to receive a recommendation for meetings of people with hypothyroidism, from an education office at your local hospital. Connecting and communicating with others who can empathize with what you are going through could end up being an enormous aid in your recovery and life with hypothyroidism.

Important as well is making sure you monitor yourself for other health conditions that could arise. As we went over earlier, the main cause for hypothyroidism is an autoimmune disease. Just as well, links with hypothyroidism have also been found in conditions such as diabetes, having pituitary issues, having your sleep obstructed by sleep apnea, and lupus.

Just as with fatigue, depression is a common symptom and side effect of going through and living with hypothyroidism and should be watched closely. The thyroid glands hormone levels lower, the function of your body begins to slow down, and before you may realize it you are living with a depression that was not there before. It is vital to know what to look out for, and not just what, but also how to look after yourself while dealing with this.

Depression as a symptom can make hypothyroidism difficult to diagnose as there are many who may only experience difficulties or changes in mood as a symptom. It is for this reason, that instead of having a doctor check only your brain when checking for depression, it can also be important to ask them to check for signs of you having an underactive thyroid. Aside from the changes in mood, there are a few other similarities that exist in both having depression as well as hypothyroidism such as, gaining weight, finding it difficult to maintain concentration, feelings of daily fatigue, which coincide with a reduced desire and satisfaction with daily life, and hypothyroidism or depression could both effect your ability to sleep well.

Not all of their symptoms overlap so nicely though, both have their conditions which differentiate one from the other. In the case of hypothyroidism there are, of course, some physical signs such as the dryness of the skin, or the thinning and loss of hair. There is also the tendency to become constipated and the increase in levels of cholesterol. These symptoms would be atypical if depression alone was the issue.

If you have hypothyroidism and it is the cause of your depression, then the correct treatment and care of the hypothyroidism should be just the remedy needed in order to treat your depression as well. If the hypothyroidism passes and depression remains, it may be important to talk to your doctor about receiving further help and a change in medication.

Along with depression being a symptom of hypothyroidism, it has recently been found, through studies, that around 60 percent or so of people who get hypothyroidism tend to also exhibit having anxiety as well. Studies are ongoing and are still growing in scope and size, though it would still be in your best interest to discuss all possibilities and symptoms with your doctor in order to more thoroughly and best tackle the treatment of hypothyroidism.

It cannot be stressed enough, how much of your body is under the affects and influence of your thyroid gland working properly to produce and secrete the correct levels of hormones. For this reason, when a woman gets hypothyroidism and simultaneously desires to get pregnant, she will be faced with her own subset of challenges to come. Have a low thyroid gland function during a pregnancy can cause a number of conflicts including various birth defects, have a still-birth or miscarriage, as well as anemia or a low birth weight. It is not uncommon for a woman with thyroid problems to have a perfectly healthy pregnancy, but to make sure that you reach this outcome it is important to do things such as eating well, keeping yourself informed about current and effective medicines, as well as talking to your doctor about testing.

Though testing may result in changes to your dosage or medication, it is also for this reason that it is important to make sure you are not deviating from the medications provided and the dosage your doctor has recommended.

Considering the thyroid issues adds on even more importance to the need for eating healthy while pregnant. Make sure that you are getting the proper amount of vitamins, minerals, and nutrients and consider taking multivitamins as well to supplement this.

It is not impossible to develop a thyroid issue such as hypothyroidism while pregnant. In fact, for every 1,000 pregnancies, this tends to occur in every 3 out of 5 women. It is important for doctors to routinely check thyroid levels during your pregnancy, as some will do, to make sure your thyroid levels aren't becoming to high or low. If they end up being higher or lower than they ought to be, it is likely that your doctor will recommend you starting treatment. Even some women who have never before had any thyroid issues may develop them once the baby is born, which is known as postpartum thyroiditis, and also tends to resolve itself after a year in around 80 percent of the women it shows up in. It is only the other 20 percent of women who will have this happen and then go on to require the long term treatment.

When hypothyroidism takes place, and the functions of the body slow down, it is quite typical for people to become prone to gaining weight, which is very likely due to what happens to the bodies ability to burn energy, which is that the efficiency to do so slows down as well. This change in the body will typically cause someone who has hypothyroidism to gain anywhere from 5 to 10 pounds in general, making the weight that is gained not entirely drastic, but someone could still find it quite alarming. It is very possible then, that once the hypothyroidism has been treated, that any weight gained will then be easily lost. If this does not occur, a simple change in diet, and adding regular exercise to your routine should aid in handily losing the weight, as your ability to manage weight will go back to normalcy, with the return to proper levels in your thyroid hormones.

Hypothyroidism is a common occurrence; therefore it is also commonly treated without issue. Hypothyroidism has been found to occur in around 4.6 percent of the American population that are 12 and older. Which comes out to about 10 million or so people who go on to live long healthy lives with the condition, and you may never even realize it. It is far more prevalent in people who are over the age of 60, and in women about 1 in 5 of them are likely to experience hypothyroidism by the time they have reached 60 years of age. One of the causes is Hashimoto's disease which happens to appear more in women who have reached middle-age, though it can absolutely show up in children and men. As Hashimoto's disease is hereditary, it is likely that if you get it, you did so from a relative, and have an increased chance then of passing it on down to your children.

It is important to keep an eye on your body, your health, and your thyroid gland as you get older. If, as the years go by, you begin to notice any of the changes gone over in this chapter so far, it is vital that you see a doctor in an attempt to get a proper diagnosis and seek treatment as soon as possible.

Hashimoto's Disease

Hashimoto's disease is an autoimmune disease which can be very destructive to your thyroid gland, and thereby your thyroid glands ability to function properly. Hashimoto's disease is also known as chronic autoimmune lymphocytic thyroiditis and is the most common cause of having an underactive thyroid gland, hypothyroidism, in the United States.

As an autoimmune disorder, Hashimoto's disease is one of many conditions that will be the cause of your body's white blood cells and your body's antibodies becoming confused and starting to attack the cells that make up the thyroid gland. What makes this happen precisely is still somewhat of a mystery to doctors, even still it is believed by some that factors of genetics may be involved.

With the cause of Hashimoto's disease being unknown, it is difficult to precisely put a finger on what puts a person at risk for having or contracting the disease. There are still, however, just a few factors that doctors are aware of which could signify being at risk for the disease. In the case of Hashimoto's disease, in particular, women happen to be seven times more likely to contract than men, and especially for women who have been pregnant before. Having a history of autoimmune diseases in the family is another factor that could mean you are at higher risk of having Hashimoto's at some point in your life, especially if the autoimmune diseases include Graves' disease, lupus, rheumatoid arthritis, if there is a history of Sjogren's syndrome in your family, or a history of type 1 diabetes, Addison's disease, and vitiligo. If it is the case that these autoimmune diseases are present in your family line or may have been based on symptoms of Hashimoto's disease, get together and discuss the possibility with your doctor, then make sure to get tested for the disease.

Hashimoto's disease is interesting in that the symptoms of it, are not symptomatic of Hashimoto's disease alone, in fact, they are similar to having the symptoms of an underactive thyroid gland, or hypothyroidism. Some signs to watch out for that your thyroid gland is not working properly to produce proper thyroid hormones, and that you may have Hashimoto's disease are your skin becoming dry and pale, constipation, if your voice becomes hoarse, you become depressed and start to feel sluggish or fatigued. High levels of cholesterol, a thinning of the hair, muscle weakness in the lower body, and intolerance to the cold may also be signs of hypothyroidism as a result of Hashimoto's disease. In women, it can also cause issues with fertility. Hashimoto's can exist inside of your body for many years before you begin to show any signs or symptoms, and during that time, it may progress while showing no signs of damage to the thyroid gland. Some with Hashimoto's disease end up with a goiter, an enlarging of the thyroid gland which causes the front of the neck to swell. Though generally painless, it is common for a goiter to make the act of swallowing difficult and for it to simulate a feeling of fullness in the throat.

Owing to it's difficulty to diagnose, your doctor may not suspect Hashimoto's of being prevalent until observing symptoms having hypothyroidism. In which case they will need to conduct a blood test designed to check the thyroid-stimulating hormone, or TSH, levels in your body. It is a relatively common and safe test, which is also an accurate way to check to see if you have Hashimoto's disease. Levels of thyroid-stimulating hormone are higher when the activity of the thyroid glad is lower because your body starts working harder to stimulate the production of more thyroid hormones to secrete from the thyroid gland. There are also blood tests that your doctor may conduct if they feel the need to check further for the levels of antibodies, cholesterol, and other thyroid hormones, T3 and T4, in your blood. Testing for all of these can help immensely in pinning down a diagnosis of Hashimoto's disease.

Unless your thyroid gland is functioning normally, in which case your doctor may still recommend regular checkups to monitor you for any changes, it is very likely that the need for treatment of Hashimoto's disease will be required.

The improper production of enough hormones in your body by your thyroid gland will likely result in the need to take medication. In the case of having to take this medication, it is also likely that you will be prescribed on it, though dose will vary, for the rest of your life. The effective drug most commonly prescribed is levothyroxine which is the hormone thyroxine, or T4, made synthetically, and which will successfully replace the missing hormone in your blood. The synthetic hormone drug levothyroxine tends not to have any noticeable side effects, and regular use has been known to frequently return the hormone levels of the body back to normal, restoring proper function of the thyroid gland. When this happens, all other symptoms of Hashimoto's disease and hypothyroidism generally tend to disappear altogether, though it is likely that your doctor will still recommend that you still get regular testing done so that your hormone levels can be consistently monitored to prevent something like hypothyroidism from becoming a problem again moving forward. Getting the regular testing allows the doctor to adjust the dosage of your medication as necessary if at all necessary.

It is important to consider before going on levothyroxine, that there are supplements and medications which will have an effect on your body's ability to absorb the drug. As such, make sure you have a discussion about this with your doctor if you are taking any other medications, especially if they include iron or calcium supplements, or estrogen. Some medications for cholesterol have been known to cause an issue, as well as proton pump inhibitors which are used as a treatment for acid reflux.

Though these have been known to cause an issue, there is what could be an easy work around of simply changing what time of the day you take your other medicines in conjunction with the doctor recommended thyroid medicine. It is also possible that certain foods could end up being involved in the efficacy of your thyroid medicine. It is best to discuss all of this with your doctor to come up with an efficient way for you to take your thyroid medicine, based on your dietary needs.

The severity of complications due to leaving Hashimoto's untreated varies and are not worth the risk if you ever contract, or if you have it. They go far beyond just hypothyroidism and include heart problems that an include total failure of the heart. It is not unusual for anemia to be a result of leaving Hashimoto's disease unattended. Depression and a decrease in libido are common, as well as higher levels of cholesterol in the blood and experiencing a sense of confusion or loss of consciousness.

Hashimoto's disease has also been the culprit responsible for complications during a woman's pregnancy cycle. It is far more likely, that if you carry out a pregnancy while having untreated Hashimoto's disease, that you may be putting your child at higher risk of being born with defects of their kidneys, their heart, and even their brains.

These complications can be limited by talking to your doctor during the pregnancy and keeping on top of monitoring your thyroid glands hormone levels with the proper blood testing. If you are a pregnant woman and have thyroid issues, such preventative measures could mean a severe change in the life and health of your child. However, if you have not had any known disorders with your thyroid or hormone levels, it is not recommended that you get regular or constant screening done during the pregnancy.

Graves' Disease

Another autoimmune disorder, Graves' disease is responsible for causing your thyroid gland too create too much of the thyroid hormones in your body. When this happens it is a condition referred to commonly as hyperthyroidism. Graves' disease, is named such for the man who discovered it, an Irish physician named Robert J. Graves, and is regarded as one of the most common forms hyperthyroidism takes, having an effect on around 1 out of every 200 people.

When Graves' disease occurs in the body, it will cause your immune system to begin creating antibodies that are known as thyroid-stimulating immunoglobulins, that attach themselves to the body's usually healthy cells of the thyroid gland. By doing this they end up causing the thyroid gland to produce and secrete more of the thyroid hormones than it is meant to for your body. The hormones that are produced by the thyroid gland go on to affect a great number of your body's functions including its temperature, the function of the nervous system, the development of the brain, and the list goes on. For this reason, hyperthyroidism can end up having a negatively driven affect on not just all of those functions, but when left untreated can also cause the loss of weight and mental and physical fatigue. Hyperthyroidism has also been found to be responsible for such things as depression and emotional liability where the individual will uncontrollably cry or laugh or put on other manic emotional displays.

Due to the role that Graves' disease can invariably play on the appearance of hyperthyroidism in the body, it is no surprise that the two would contain a sharing of many of the same symptoms. These symptoms include tremors especially of the hands, a loss of weight, tachycardia, which is the rapidity in the rate of the heart, becoming intolerant to heat or warmth, fatigue, nervousness and irritability, the swelling of the front of the neck, due to the enlargement of the thyroid gland, known as a goiter, an increase in the frequency of having bowel movements, as well as diarrhea, weakness of the muscles, and having it become difficult to get a good full night's worth of sleep. Among the people who experience having Graves' disease, it is only a small percentage who will experience the skin thickening around their shin area and become reddened, an affliction which is known as Graves' dermopathy.

Another common symptom of Graves' disease which one may go through while experiencing the condition, is what is called Graves' ophthalmopathy. Graves' ophthalmopathy is what occurs when the eyes of the afflicted individual appear to be enlarged, which is a result of the eyelids retracting. When Graves' ophthalmopathy happens, it is entirely possible that your eyes may begin to bulge outwards from your eye sockets. Estimates say that as much as 30 percent of the people who end up developing Graves' disease will observe at least a mild case of what is known as Graves' ophthalmopathy and that for up to 5 percent of the people will instead experience an extreme case of the eye bulging.

Because of autoimmune diseases such as Graves' disease, the immune system will begin to fight against what are the healthy cells and healthy tissues of the body. Normally, your immune system is producing proteins which are known as antibodies, which are responsible for fighting against foreign invaders to your body, the likes of harmful viruses and bacteria. The antibodies produced this way are formed especially with the duty of targeting a specific invader to the host. When it comes to the effect of Graves' disease on the body, your immune system begins to mistake healthy thyroid cells as these foreign harmful cells and produces the thyroid-stimulating immunoglobulins which then mistakenly go off to attack what are your healthy thyroid cells.

Scientists and doctors alike, are aware that it is indeed possible for a person to have inherited the ability for their body to make antibodies which then go against their own healthy cells, yet they have made no determination that such an occurrence is what is the cause for Graves' disease, or who will end up developing Graves' disease.

Despite that though, there are experts who believe that they have been able to button down on some factors which may increase ones risk for the development of graves disease which includes its tendency to be hereditary. So be sure to discuss family medical history with your doctor and talk about whether or not there are family members who have, or who ay have had Graves' disease. It is also believed by these experts that stress, gender, and someone's age may be some of the facets that end up putting someone at higher risk of getting Graves' disease. It is typical for the disease to be found in people who are younger than the age of 40, and it has been more prevalent, about seven to eight times so, in women rather than men.

Having had, or having still, another autoimmune disease is yet another factor that will increase your risk of ever getting Graves' disease. Examples of such autoimmune diseases are having Crohn's disease, rheumatoid arthritis, and diabetes mellitus, among others.

For the diagnosing of Graves' disease, when it is suspected, it is not unheard of for your doctor to request lab tests. The use of your families medical history as well, especially if there is a case of someone in your family having had Graves' disease, will be able to help act as a basis for your doctor to zero in on diagnosing whether you have Graves' disease as well or not. This is something that thyroid gland blood tests will be needed for in order to confirm. Your doctor may request that these tests and others may be handled by a specialist expert in diseases which are related to the body's hormones, known as an endocrinologist, in order to help get the diagnosis of Graves' disease. Other tests which your doctor may request are full bloodwork tests, a thyroid gland scan, an uptake test utilizing radioactive iodine, a test for levels of TSH, or thyroid stimulating hormone, and a TSI test, which is the thyroid-stimulating immunoglobulins.

By combining the efforts of the endocrinologist, as well as the array of tests, it is more possible for your doctor to determine if you do indeed have and need treatment for Graves' disease specifically, or if another thyroid disorder is what is at work, and thus requires its own specific form of treatment.

There are a number of options available for treatment when someone is diagnosed as having Graves' disease. These are generally the taking of anti-thyroid drugs, therapy in the form of RAI, or radioactive iodine, and getting thyroid gland surgery. It is not abnormal for a doctor, in the case of Graves' disease, to recommend, all, two, or just one of the treatments for the afflicted.

When it comes to treatment via anti-thyroid drugs, you will typically be taking medications such as methimazole, which is taken orally as a tablet and works by putting a stop to the thyroid gland producing and secreting too much thyroid hormone, and propylthiouracil, which is also taken orally and generally used as a back up if a drug like methimazole did not end up working well enough. The use of beta-blockers is also recommended on occasion as they are used in assistance of reducing the effects of symptoms until another treatment method can start working.

It is radioactive iodine treatment, or RAI, which is among the most common treatments suggested to those suffering of Graves' disease. It is required, during this treatment, that the individual seeking treatment take specified doses of radioactive iodine-131, the purpose of which is to destroy thyroid cells. The radioactive iodine-131 will be ingested orally, in small amounts, via pill. Be sure to discuss with your doctor and risks or precautions that come with this treatment.

The less frequent option for treatment is the thyroid surgery. This treatment will tend to be a last resort if the other options have not worked to full capacity, if there is a reason to be suspect of thyroid cancer being present, or if the patient is a pregnant woman who is unable to take any of the regularly prescribed anti-thyroid drugs.

In the case of surgery being necessary, it is not uncommon the doctor to issue the removal of your thyroid gland completely, in the interest of preventing the return of the hyperthyroidism. In which case, thyroid hormone replacement surgery will be necessary on a regular basis. Talk to your doctor about the possible side effects of choosing to go through with surgery, as well as generally what to expect moving forward.

Goiter

A goiter, goitre, thyroid cyst, or Plummer's disease, is a general term used for when there is an observable enlargement of the thyroid gland, usually resulting in a noticeable swelling of the front of the neck. Treatment for a goiter can be handled in a variety of ways, and the treatment method is dependent on the goiters location, the length of its presence, and how exactly it is affecting the thyroid glands performance.

Though usually unable to be seen or even felt, the thyroid gland generally tends to become detectable by touch and even perceptible to the eye when there is a goiter present. An expanse of the thyroid gland, or goiter, can be the cause of the whole thyroid gland expanding, which is known as a "smooth goiter", or just a part of the thyroid gland expanding, which is also called a "cystic" or "nodular" goiter. A goiter is not a sure symptom of having an active thyroid, known as hyperthyroidism, or underactive thyroid, known as hypothyroidism, and, in fact, the majority of people who have a goiter, retain a perfectly normal use of their thyroid gland.

A number of reasons exist for the existence of a goiter. Among these are included a deficiency in your levels of iodine. Iodine may be a trace element, but it is far from trivial. It assists in helping the thyroid gland in maintaining proper functionality and making the thyroid glands hormones. There are two primary hormones which are produced and secreted by the thyroid gland, these are T4 or thyroxine, and T3, also known as triiodothyronine. The approximate number of people who have iodine deficiency comes out to about 2.2 billion and it is estimated that around 29 percent of the worlds total population live in an area that is considered to be deficient in iodine. It is reported that people in the U.K. have proper levels of iodine as a part of their regular diet. If you are keeping your eye out for food sources that are a good source of iodine, there are salts that have iodine supplements, as well, non-organic milk is plentiful with iodine.

Thyroiditis is anther well known cause of goiter. Thyroiditis is more commonly referred to as when the thyroid gland has become inflamed. Around the world, the most common reason for thyroiditis occurring is Hashimoto's disease, or Hashimoto's thyroiditis, which is an autoimmune disease that causes the bodies antibodies to start to become confused and begin attacking healthy cells of the thyroid gland. Hashimoto's disease is not the only cause of the thyroiditis condition though, it could also stem from viral infection, and has been known to occur just after or during pregnancy.

A goiter has also been known to occur due to Graves' disease, another autoimmune disease, this one causing the immune systems antibodies attacks on thyroid cells to make the thyroid gland overactive, resulting in hyperthyroidism. It is this hyperthyroidism, or over activity of the thyroid glands capacity for producing and secreting hormones, which is the cause of the swelling of the thyroid gland.

If there are benign growths on the thyroid gland, they have been known to cause a goiter, most commonly known for doing this is a follicular adenoma, which can be a firm or rubbery tumor surrounded by a fibrous capsule.

External factors that may be the cause of goiter are known as goitrogens. Included among what would be considered a goitrogen are medicines such as the mental health drug lithium, and cabbage type vegetables. Ingestion in the excess of these vegetables, which include cassava or kelp, will likely result in the growth formation of a goiter.

There are physiological demands put on the body during pregnancy and during puberty which have been known to be at the root of a goiter. And as with other causes like Graves' disease and Hashimoto's disease, there is a strong likelihood of inherited genetic reasons that one may at some point experience goiter.

Due to the varying reasons for the existence of goiter, there are also a multiplicity of types of goiter. The first of these types is known as colloid goiter, or endemic goiter, which is a development due directly to a lack of sufficient iodine levels. As a result, the people who tend to end up with a colloid goiter are those we mentioned, who live somewhere with a less dense supply of iodine.

The next type of goiter is the nontoxic goiter, or sporadic goiter, as it is also well known. Though the definite cause of a goiter of this type is regarded as generally unknown, it is surmised that a sporadic goiter is a result of taking medications, such as lithium, for example, or so it is believed. Among the may uses for lithium, it is perhaps most commonly recognized as the drug used for aiding in the treatment of mood based disorders, the likes of bipolar or depression. The nontoxic name is apt in regard to this form of goiter, as they are benign, and have no discernable effect on the production or secretion function of the thyroid gland, leaving the thyroid to function at a healthy and normal capacity.

The final type of commonly recognized goiter is known as the toxic nodular or multinodular goiter. Generally originating and taking form from as merely an extension from what was a simple goiter prior, the toxic nodular goiter will take the form of at least one, but often more, small nodules on the expanding thyroid gland. This toxic nodular goiter, having taken a sort of root on the thyroid gland, then begins to produce its own thyroid hormone, which plays a big part in the causation of hyperthyroidism.

As mentioned above, it can be difficult to detect goiter before it has really taken effect to the thyroid gland, but after it has begun doing it's work it is most common for it to cause a swelling of the front of the neck, making it clearly visible as well as felt. Before the expanding has commenced, it is common to have had nodules existing in your thyroid gland, these small nodules cannot be felt, and may have even been only a chance occurrence due to examinations, and of scans, that were applied for other reasons. Cases such as these are rather common, and when they occur, there has been a tendency to notice no sign of a goiter up to that point. As nodules appear on the thyroid, ranging from smaller nodules to much larger nodules, it is the presence of these nodules which is what is the cause of noticeable swelling of the neck.

This swelling and the nodules which are collecting on the thyroid gland cause other symptoms to occur, like having a difficult time of swallowing or of trying to breathe, it is not uncommon for coughing to be a symptom, your voice may start to become hoarse, and there may be a dizzy sensation that is noticeable when you raise an arm above your head.

Goiter is a rather common occurrence. It is calculated by the World Health Organization, that around the world, goiter affects nearly 12 percent of the global population. However, it has also been recorded that in Europe, the rate of goiter is lower by a slight amount. Goiter being considered endemic, or noticeably affecting a certain area is a common occurrence wherever iodine is scarce, and the endemic definitions are only applied when goiter is recognized on 1 out of 10 people within a certain population.

It is usual for goiter to be the diagnosis when there is noticeable swelling on the neck that can be seen without the need of a scan, also making it detectable with the touch of the hand, due to the enlarged thyroid gland in your neck, something a doctor will be quick to check for, likely before anything else.

There are also a number tests a general practitioner may order in order to examine the levels in your blood of thyroid hormones coming from the thyroid gland, as well as wanting to make sure of the levels of antibodies that are prevalent in the bloodstream. This examination will often take the form of blood tests, that are used to detect the changes in levels of the hormones as well as whether or not the level of production of the antibodies has increased, which tends to happen in response to the body experiencing an injury or infection in the blood.

A thyroid scan, or thyroid uptake scan, will show the size of the goiter itself, as well as what condition the goiter is in. It will also aid in identifying any differences in activity, in various places on the thyroid gland.

A biopsy may be recommended, the procedure of which involves removing samples of your thyroid gland, and then sending the samples of your thyroid gland's tissue to an outside laboratory or endocrinologist for examination.

It is also possible that an ultrasound scan may be used which will help for a doctor to see images of the inside of your neck, getting a much closer look at the size of the invasive goiter, allowing for the observation of nodules. As more ultrasounds are done, it is even then possible to track the changes in size or shape of the nodules, and the size of the goiter.

You may, at some point, be referred to an endocrinologist in order to get an outpatient assessment, giving you and the doctor more information from the examination by an expert. During their examination you may have to undergo a test known as a fine needle aspiration, which is done on the thyroid gland. For the procedure to take place, the endocrinologist will make use of a fine needle which, utilizing the guiding sight of an ultrasound, will be used to remove tissue from your thyroid gland, only a small amount will be needed. The tissue removed from your thyroid gland is then studied under the lens of a microscope, which will assist the endocrinologist in assessing exactly the types of cells which are currently present in your thyroid gland. It is not at all uncommon for a procedure like this to need to be repeated one or more times, for the sake of reaching an accurate result and helping you on your way to treatment and recovery.

There is no one, cut and dry, blanket method for treating a goiter, as the treatment will depend entirely on precisely what is the cause that is underlying the goiter. As well, a particular course of action will be decided by your doctor on the basis of the size of the goiter, and the condition that the goiter is in, as well as the symptoms you have that are associated with the goiter. It will also be important to not overlook any factors to your health that may have been responsible for the goiters formation when looking into treatment options.

A goiter which can be regarded as simple, having a prevalence of causing no imbalances in the thyroid gland, as well as no seeming problems as a result of the thyroid gland, will be less likely to cause further obstructions or overall issues.

In order to shrink a goiter, in the case of hypo or hyperthyroidism, it may be enough to just take prescribed medicines as a treatment for the symptoms and for the swelling of the thyroid gland. Medications which are known as corticosteroids often see use in the task of reducing any inflammation, or when there is a prevalence of thyroiditis.

Medicinal treatments for a goiter are not always the most effective response, however. It is not at all uncommon for a goiter to have grown too large to be able to respond properly to medicinal therapy and begin to shrink. In such a case there are surgeries which are available, known as a thyroidectomy. Undergoing a thyroidectomy will mean removing your thyroid gland completely and is a common option for when the thyroid gland grows too large and further obstructs what would otherwise be simple actions, such as swallowing or breathing.

When you are going through the experience of trying to treat what is the most harmful of the goiter family, the toxic nodular or multinodular goiter, RAI, or radioactive iodine treatment is typically the necessary response. You will be given a tablet, the RAI, which is a small amount of the radioactive iodine, which gets ingested orally and begins the process of destroying thyroid gland tissue.

When it comes to the treatment of a goiter, there are options for home care which can be very helpful and ought not to be overlooked as such. When you have finished up with all the treatment that can be offered at the hospital, or by a referred endocrinologist, it is an entirely common possibility that a discussion with your general practitioner will end in him or her suggesting you continue care of yourself in the home, with a prescription of some form of medication, which may end up being a decrease or increase in the amounts of iodine that you are ingesting regularly. This will, of course, be determined by the type of goiter that was ailing you, as well as requiring regular testing to keep an eye on your iodine levels, and the efficiency of your thyroid glands production and secretion of hormones. If it all ends up that a goiter is non-problematic, being too small to count as an issue or cause an imbalance, you may require no treatment or care at home at all.

Conclusion

The next step is to begin implementing the various methods of relief repented within this book so that you can immediately address the symptoms of acid reflux before they take root. Addressing the symptoms, in this manner, will allow your body to fight off disease like GERD and Barrett's disease as soon as possible rather than at a later time when your body is significantly weaker. Keep in mind that the best method of addressing your symptoms is to consult a medical professional. In this way, you can begin to implement the strategies presented in this book with guidance from a qualified medical professional.

Given that your acid reflux is likely to exist on a ranging spectrum and will most definitely be different for every individual, this book provides methods of addressing your symptoms and ailments in a manner that is applicable and helpful for whichever stage of the reflux you are experiencing. What's more, the 30-day recovery plan is a great way to ensure that your symptoms are staved off for good once you can utilize medical intervention. If, for instance, you are prescribed drugs to mitigate your symptoms, be sure to use the methods outlined in this book in conjunction with the prescribed amount of medication that your doctor has instructed.

Where your health is concerned, being prepared and informed is critical to seeing that you successfully overcome the ailments that are affecting you.

That is precisely why this book is of value. After reading, you are now informed about the intricate aspects of acid reflux and should feel extremely prepared as you move forward in addressing these symptoms.

For this is not truly the end is it, but merely a small step in a forward direction. It is now time to utilize what you have learned going through these pages, and all that the knowledge contained within has to offer. If you or a loved one you know has, has had, or may seem to have a thyroid issue, every tool that is needed to aid them or yourself in the journey forward is now at your fingertips.

Now is when it is time to go see a doctor, to make sure that information is properly communicated. It is never too late, and never a bad idea, especially where the thyroid gland is concerned, to set oneself up with a regular and balanced diet, as well as having a plan for daily exercise in a range of activities.

CPSIA information can be obtained
at www.ICGtesting.com
Printed in the USA
FSHW012025220520
70536FS

9 781913 710095